FROM PREMENSTRUAL SYNDROME TO POSTPARTUM DEPRESSION: UNDERSTANDING THE PHASES OF A WOMAN'S BODY

ANIBABA OMOYEMI

DEDICATION.

This book is dedicated to every woman who at different stages in life will undergo various changes in their bodies. From a girl child to a lady, then to womanhood and finally menopausal.

Table of Contents

ACKNOWLEDGMENTS.

Foremost, I acknowledge and reverence the Holy Spirit for divine inspiration. Also, I acknowledge Oluwatobi Salako, my husband for motivation and my sister, Anibaba Titilayo nee Odetola, for inspiring me to put this piece together. Thank you and God bless.

Introduction

Most people, especially women, have a mystery about the female body! When discussing the who, what, when, where, and why of the female anatomy, people naturally become a little perplexed because of cycles and stages, hot flashes, and periods. This book ought to shed some light on the situation. After finishing this article, you should have a newfound appreciation for the intricate systems that maintain the health of our bodies. If not, at least you'll be aware of the precise reasons for Premenstrual Syndrome and morning sickness in pregnant women.

Are you prepared to learn everything there is to know about female physiology? Hold on firmly. It'll be a sentimental, queasy, and otherwise stereotypically female ride.

Please note: This book is not a substitute for medical advice. If you have any conditions or complaints, they should be checked out by a licensed physician. The content included herein is for informational purposes only.

Chapter 1- Once Again, It's That Time of the Month.

You might hear a lot about it. The rag, Aunt Flow, or that time of the month are all terms used by women. All of these creative names are used to describe the same thing: menstruation.

Menstruation

Menstruation, sometimes known as one's "period," happens every 28 days on average. A young girl will experience her first period starting around the age of 12, although a little before or a bit later is completely natural. Until she becomes pregnant or until she hits menopause later in life, she will have a period roughly every

month.

However, during these 28 days, there is always something going on in a woman's reproductive system. The menstrual cycle takes about 28 days to complete and takes in several stages. For convenience's sake, we've divided the cycle into two halves.

Menstrual Cycle Part 1

The body starts preparing for the chance of becoming pregnant at the start of the menstrual cycle. As a result, the body begins thickening the uterine lining as estrogen levels rise. The egg or ovum is stimulated to mature in one of the ovaries at the same time.

Ovulation, or the release of the developed egg from the ovary, occurs midway during this period.

Menstrual Cycle Part 2

The egg starts to travel via the fallopian tube after being expelled from the ovary. A woman can become pregnant at this period. If the egg is fertilized, it will attach itself to the lining when the uterine lining is at its thickest, and pregnancy will start. If the egg is not fertilized, it is expelled from the body during menstruation along with the uterine lining. Through the cervix and the vagina, this substance is expelled from the body.

Dealing With The Period

When people talk about a woman's menstruation, the rule of averages is in operation. The truth is that no two women are precisely the same. A woman may experience a period that lasts two days which is extremely painful, while another woman may experience a period that lasts eight days which is moderately painful, with moderate bleeding. It's really difficult to predict one's experience.

However, in terms of averages, a period often lasts three to five days. Some women find that taking over-the-counter medication is necessary to lessen period discomfort.
As a teen, one's period might be somewhat unpredictable and irregular, which just adds to the enjoyment of the already stressful teen years. As a woman ages, her cycle should become more predictable and regular. If this is not the case, birth control tablets are frequently advised to keep things on a regular and healthy schedule.

There are two ways for menstruation women to control their menstrual flow. These are either sanitary napkins or tampons and pads.

Common Menstrual Problems

As you might anticipate, a woman's menstrual cycle is not all fun and games. Even though they are generally handled without too many problems, menstruation troubles are widespread and impact many women (except cramps and PMS, of course).

Dysmenorrhea

Dysmenorrhea is essentially a condition characterized by painful periods. Intense menstrual cramps are usually the most prevalent symptom. Occasionally, an underlying ailment can cause pain.

Endometriosis is a painful condition that results in the growth of uterine tissue in other areas of the body. During menstruation, this swollen tissue has nowhere to go, which can cause intense anguish. Long-term effects of this condition could include infertility, irregular periods, and sex pain.

Fibroids, which are benign tumors, adhere to the uterine wall. They could lead to painful menstrual cycles, excessive bleeding, and possibly infertility.

Amenorrhea

The absence of a period is this situation. A woman's period may have never begun, or it may have begun and abruptly stopped for her. Amenorrhea can have many different causes, depending on the person, but they can range from difficulties from an eating disorder, stress, or exercise, to pregnancy and breastfeeding.

Menorrhagia

Menorrhagia is essentially abnormal vaginal or uterine bleeding. It might manifest as very heavy bleeding, very long periods, menstruation every other week, or bleeding between cycles that is considerably heavier than spotting. Women who are on the verge of menopause or who are experiencing hormonal issues frequently get this illness.

Period Abnormalities

As previously said, the majority of women start having periods between the ages of 11 and 15.This is entirely typical. But if a woman is 16 years old and has not yet experienced menstruation, she should visit a doctor. Other menstrual-related causes for seeing a doctor include:
- Prolonged bleeding
- Severe cramping in the abdomen.
- A time frame that is significantly longer than usual.
- Bleeding between periods that is more severe than spotting.
- A phase that ended unexpectedly.

Toxic Shock Syndrome

Tampon use can result in a disorder known as toxic shock syndrome, or TSS. TSS can be fatal, so it's critical to understand the warning signs, symptoms, and steps you can take to avoid it.

Symptoms

- A high fever

- Diarrhea.

- Red, swollen eyes.

- Acute vertigo.

- Muscle aches.

- Rash.

- A sore throat

Preventative Measures

Pay close attention to the directions on the tampon pack in order to help prevent the possibly fatal TSS. Tampons should only be used during periods. Consider your own flow and use the least amount of absorbency required. Tampons should be changed frequently rather than left in for extended periods of time. Finally, consider switching between pads and tampons every 4 to 8 hours, especially on your light days.

Chapter 2 – Premenstrual Syndrome (PMS) Is Not Just "Cramps"

Oh, PMS, or more specifically Premenstrual Syndrome, is the bane of most women's lives.

Can you believe that once, people thought PMS was a myth? On the contrary, many women experience it every month and it is a real condition with actual symptoms.

These signs start approximately a week before your period begins and typically go away as soon as menstruation starts. However, many women also suffer PMS during their menstruation and up to 14 days before it.

The discomfort you experience before your period and PMS are not the same thing. Due to physical discomfort or mental turbulence, PMS makes it practically difficult to perform at work or at home.

Causes of PMS

Although the exact origin of PMS is unknown, the hormonal changes and variations that occur at specific times during a woman's menstrual cycle are most likely to be to blame. It's critical to understand that PMS is not brought on by any underlying psychological issue. Instead, anxiety and difficult circumstances could make PMS symptoms worse.

Symptoms of PMS

There are many different PMS symptoms. Have you figured it out yet? Every aspect of the processes that take place in the female body differs across different women. However, a few of the most typical PMS signs are as follows:

- A bigger appetite.
- Depression.
- Constipation.
- Bloating.
– Edema or swollen limbs.
- Joint and muscle soreness.
- Anxiety and irritability.
- A decrease in sex urge.
- Problems with sleep.
- Soft breasts.
- Tiredness.
- Headaches.
- A hard time focusing.

PMS Treatments

Although PMS cannot be cured, there are several strategies to treat and manage it. There are numerous things you can do at home to control PMS (see the section below), but if your doctor feels that medication is essential to appropriately treat your symptoms, then they can be prescribed.

Antidepressants

Antidepressant medications may be recommended to some women who have significant anxiety, nervousness, and irritability as a result of PMS in order to assist control the mood swings that would otherwise be raging due to hormonal changes.

Diuretics

Diuretics, which aid in the body's elimination of surplus salt and fluid—the main causes of PMS bloat—are commonly referred to as "water pills." You'll typically be recommended to start taking the diuretic pills right before the onset of your PMS symptoms after carefully monitoring your symptoms.

Birth Control Pills

The Pill's ability to lessen the severity of hormone fluctuations can significantly aid in stabilizing PMS symptoms. There is evidence that some women's periods can become less painful and shorter when taking birth control pills. However, birth control has hazards of its own and should be thought about before opting to take it, just like any other medicine.

Home Remedies

We've spoken about what your doctor can do to assist you get rid of those annoying PMS symptoms; now let's look at what you can do at home.
Of course, there are a number of over-the-counter drugs that can be used to treat PMS and other issues associated to periods. Usually, they mix a diuretic with an analgesic. However, there are other things you may do to lessen how uncomfortable your period is.

- **Eat Healthily**. Starting with a healthy diet, PMS symptoms might be lessened. To lessen irritation, stay away from foods high in sugar and fat, and attempt to completely cut off caffeine. Additionally, consuming a lot of salt can significantly increase bloat. Try to limit your intake of salt in the days before to your monthly flow. Finally, split up those big dinners. It can be difficult on the stomach to eat three full meals a day, which can result in constipation, bloating, and a variety of other PMS-related issues. Try eating six small meals rather than three large ones.

- **Sleep soundly**. An effort should be made to maintain a consistent bedtime and wake-up time. Try to obtain eight hours of sleep every night. Establish your bed as a place for relaxation, not for everything else you might do, such eating, reading, watching TV, or working!

    - **Exercise sensibly**. Try regularly exercising every other day. At least 30 minutes of aerobic exercise should be completed four times each week. - Schedule correctly. Even though certain things cannot be changed, make an effort to move stressful events and occurrences to the week after your period. Your stress level and overall discomfort are reduced as a result.

Taking in plenty of calcium is a fantastic additional defense against PMS. A daily dose of 1000 mg helps to lessen the bloating, cramping, and joint discomfort brought on by your next menstruation. Additionally, you can't overlook the other fantastic advantages of a consistent calcium diet, such as strong bones and teeth as well as a lower risk of developing osteoporosis in later life.

Your PMS may be hardly evident during other months. Others might find it impossible to control. It is crucial to understand the functions and phases that women experience as well as how we may make each of them simpler to manage because the female body can be extremely unpredictable.

Chapter 3 – Pregnancy

Pregnancy is one of the most happy and challenging moments in a woman's life. It is lovely, yet physically demanding and nerve-wracking. This section explains the conception process in detail as well as fertility problems, how to detect pregnancy, and what to expect along the journey.

Fertility and Conception

Some people suddenly become pregnant, while others have to put a lot of effort into getting pregnant. Much of it relies on where you are in life and if you are naturally predisposed to being pregnant.

Preconception

To make sure you try to conceive on the best days, there are several ways to keep an eye on your fertility. Your basal body temperature, often known as your BBT, can be tracked using one of the most used methods. A woman's BBT, which measures her body temperature while she is at rest, might reveal a lot about her cycle and fertility. This can be accomplished by taking your temperature each morning when you get up at the same time with a digital thermometer. Record the temperature every morning starting on the day you start your period.

You will experience a.4-degree increase in body temperature following ovulation. You now understand that your most fertile days—the ideal time to try to get pregnant—were the days before this rise in temperature. Charting the cervical fluid is another technique to keep an eye on your fertility. Before urinating, you can accomplish this by wiping the vaginal area with your fingers. The fluid will have the consistency of egg white, be a little transparent, moist, and stretchy if you are ovulating. Given that this type of cervical fluid indicates peak fertility, this is the ideal moment to engage in sexual activity. There is a time of creamy, white fluid before and after this phase. This is your body's natural method of letting you know when you're ready to conceive, despite the fact that it may seem a little nasty.

Boosting Fertility

Not every couple is able to conceive a baby in that manner. In truth, many women need to increase their fertility by keeping an eye on their everyday habits. An individual's capacity to conceive is influenced by their ability to maintain a healthy weight, eat sensibly, and exercise frequently. While women should focus on maintaining a healthy weight, men should also be aware of this requirement.

In addition to overall health, the foods you eat can significantly influence fertility. Include the following foods in your diet:

- **Antioxidants:** Green tea, in particular, is a fantastic source of antioxidants that support a strong immune system and guarantee a healthy pregnancy.

- **Vitamin C**: Citrus fruits, such as oranges, are excellent for boosting fertility.

- Water: Drinking your recommended eight 8 to 8 ounce glasses of water each day can have a significant positive impact on fertility.

- **Calcium**: For a healthy pregnancy and childbirth, women in particular need a lot of calcium. After all, it encourages the development of strong bones.

- **Folic Acid**: Whole grains and green, leafy veggies are excellent for both you and your unborn child. Birth deformities can be prevented by eating food rich in folic acid.

Fertility Problems

Infertility affects many couples, where one or both partners have a disease that makes it difficult for them to conceive.

Infertility may result from:

Ovulation issues.

Lack of sperm.

Sperm of low quality.

Cervical, vaginal, and other reproductive organ infections.

A few ailments, including diabetes.

STDs.

Aging.

Radiation exposure from sources such as cancer treatments.

Genetic conditions.

As you can see, a number of factors affect a couple's ability to become pregnant. Infertility can be brought on by a single issue, but the majority of couples who experience reproductive issues deal with multiple issues. Consult your doctor for the best treatment options for reproductive problems. It may be time to visit the doctor so both men and women can be tested if you have been trying to get pregnant for a year without success.

Signs and Signals of Pregnancy

You might occasionally only have a sneaking suspicion that you're pregnant, not even because you omitted a period. Instead, the body gives out multiple signs of pregnancy weeks before a pregnancy test can even show a result. If you've been trying to conceive and have noticed one or more of the signs listed below, you might already be pregnant!

Light Spotting: Spotting at the beginning of pregnancy is totally normal and shows that the egg has successfully inserted itself in the uterine lining. Mild cramping could result from this.

Tender Breasts: Your breasts will start to grow and feel larger in the early stages of pregnancy. They might also feel strangely tender, painful, or both.

Nausea: Morning sickness can occur as early as two weeks after conception, although it usually doesn't until approximately four weeks. In particular after eating or when exposed to strong odors, you may feel queasy and vomit.

Fatigue: Early in pregnancy, your body is getting ready to support and care for the life that is developing inside of you. Your body creates extra blood to meet the carrying of nutrients to the baby, which causes your heart to beat more quickly. You're going to feel exhausted after doing all of this inside effort..

Dizziness: During the first trimester of pregnancy, a variety of causes may contribute to dizziness. As your body's blood arteries enlarge to handle the increased blood flow, your blood pressure decreases. This feeling of dizziness may also be caused by low blood sugar.

Constipation: Exhaustion is a typical pregnant symptom. Funny thing is, weariness affects more than simply how you feel and behave. Additionally, the digestive system is slowed. High levels of the hormone progesterone might cause constipation because they slow down digestion.

Cravings and Aversion: Pregnant women are renowned for having an acute sense of smell. Little do people realize that women's severely bad reactions to some foods are actually caused by their increased olfactory awareness. Coffee, spicy foods, meats, and dairy products are the main offenders. Additionally, pregnant women are renowned for having bizarre desires. Early in pregnancy, your food genuinely tastes different because your hormones are preparing your body to develop a human being.

Elevated Basal Body Temperature: Your basal body temperature, also known as BBT, is the temperature you are at when you first wake up in the morning. Because the BBT is somewhat elevated at this stage of the cycle, many women utilize it to track their ovulation. You are likely pregnant if your BBT remains elevated for two weeks or more after ovulation.

Every stage of your pregnancy has its own set of difficulties. As your body changes, so will your expectations of both yourself and other people. The information that follows explains what to expect during each trimester of your pregnancy as well as how to keep your mind, body, and soul healthy for the unborn child.

First Trimester

That's it! A tiny baby is starting to develop inside of you, and you may not even be aware that you are pregnant. However, getting pregnant causes profound alterations. Being pregnant is one of the most physically taxing experiences a woman can go through, so it doesn't hurt to review some of the fundamentals.

Symptoms

The majority of the symptoms you'll experience in the first trimester of pregnancy are the same as or closely related to those that may have first indicated you were expecting. You may experience nausea, dizziness, exhaustion, aching breasts, and frequent urination as hormones start to flood your body in preparation for a brand-new life. Although dealing with these symptoms can be challenging, with a little information you can handle these pregnancy afflictions like an expert.

For instance, eating smaller meals, keeping saltines close by, and avoiding smells that make you uncomfortable can help to alleviate nausea if you're experiencing morning sickness. Alternatively, if you feel dizzy when standing still for an extended amount of time, rise up from a nap or from sitting gently. You can learn to manage with these early pregnancy symptoms, even though they might initially seem impossible to handle pregnancy test.

Prenatal Exam

The first item on your pregnant to-do list should be this. The first thing you should do after learning you are pregnant is to schedule an appointment with your healthcare provider, even if you might want to go shopping for adorable items to decorate the nursery. During this initial appointment, a lot of information about you, your health, and your unborn child will be covered. Consider going through all that follows:

A health evaluation: Basically, a routine physical exam will be performed on you to assess your general health. Get prepared to be weighed, have your height measured, and have your heart examined.

Medical Background. The doctor will ask you questions this time with your pregnancy in mind, which is annoying because it seems like you are asked the same questions every time you visit. Your menstrual cycle, allergies, and family history of specific medical concerns, such as genetic flaws, will all be questioned.

Pelvic Examination: Your doctor will check for any abnormalities in the cervix and vagina. They'll also check to see how far along you are in your pregnancy.

Blood Tests: Blood tests are essential necessary in order to record vital information about you, even though nobody enjoys needles. They will perform tests to determine your blood type, Rh factor, and history of exposure to illnesses like syphilis, measles, and hepatitis B.

Urinalysis Samples: Yes, you must urinate into a cup. However, this test is useful for figuring out whether you have a kidney or bladder infection as well as if you qualify for gestational diabetes.

Due Date: Your due date is one of the most significant things you'll learn at your prenatal exam! You may find this by taking the day of your most recent menstruation and multiplying it by 40 weeks.

Diet and Exercise

As soon as you learn you're pregnant, a prenatal vitamin should become a regular part of your routine. You should immediately stop smoking, and you should also stop drinking alcohol. Keep in mind that whatever you put into your body, you also put into the body of your unborn child.

You should be able to continue your usual exercise program with the approval of your doctor. If you don't like to exercise, start walking. This will assist you in maintaining a healthy weight during your pregnancy and help you stay strong for labor and delivery.

Development

You may be wondering at this point what the kid is doing inside the womb while you continue to visit the doctor and throw up frequently. The first three months of your baby's existence are known as the first trimester. Let's examine it week by week.

Pregnancy is focused on during weeks 1-3: They consist of your most recent period, conception, and the precise moment the fertilized egg implants itself in the uterus.

Weeks 4-6: The baby becomes an embryo at week 4 and starts to develop the brain and spinal cord, among other important organ systems. Week 5 sees your baby's first heartbeats and the first indication of face features appears in Week 6.

Weeks 7-9: Your baby's development during these three weeks is marked by the appearance of the umbilical cord, finished limbs, fingers, and toes, as well as the first indications of movement. Although the baby might start moving as early as week 9, you won't be able to feel it just yet.

Weeks 10–12: At week 10, the embryonic tail vanishes and the development of the bones starts. At week 11, the child is recognized as a fetus, and its sex may now be easily ascertained. At week 12, the baby's fingernails and toenails start to grow to a length of up to three inches. Second Trimester

Second Trimester

Moving along quickly! The second trimester of pregnancy is regarded by many women as being the most joyful. By this point, most of the morning sickness and lethargy have passed, and the baby is still not big enough to feel like it is squashing your internal organs and making you terribly uncomfortable. Take advantage of these three months while you can!

Symptoms

Many of the physical signs and symptoms that occur during the second trimester of pregnancy are understandable, but they should still be noted. After all, it's always better to be prepared.

The Protruding Belly: It makes sense that your belly expands! In fact, up until the time of delivery, you'll typically gain about 4 pounds per month. Your uterus expands as your child does. Your abdomen grows together with the size of your uterus.

Larger Breasts: Did you know that during pregnancy, your breasts might enlarge by up to two cup sizes? The glands that make milk in your breasts are stimulated by the hormones raging through your body. The breasts can also develop fat deposits.

Constipation: This might have been an issue for you in the first trimester as well, but it can continue to be a problem for the remainder of your pregnancy. Your baby's growth puts pressure on your internal organs, slowing down the digestive process and leading to issues like constipation.

Vaginal discharge: A little bit more discharge during the second trimester is quite acceptable. This extremely acidic discharge is thought to aid in warding off microorganisms that could potentially enter the vagina.

Braxton-Hicks: These contractions might be thought of as "practice" contractions. Your uterus begins to fortify itself early since it has a huge task to complete on delivery day. Lower abdominal and groin contractions that are painless are entirely typical.

Bladder Infections: You are more prone to get a bladder infection the longer pee stays in your bladder. The bladder is compressed as the uterus expands, slowing the flow of pee even further. In order to counteract this unfavorable side effect, make sure to drink lots of water.

Dizziness and Shortness of Breath: Your body expands blood vessels in preparation for the baby, but there may not be enough blood to fill them, which can make you feel lightheaded. Although this issue usually resolves itself, it's advised to avoid standing for extended periods of time to prevent dizziness. Similar to how your lungs are absorbing more oxygen than ever before, you are beginning to feel a little short of breath.

Darkened Skin: As a result of all of this increased blood flow, your skin's pigment might also alter, particularly on your face, genital region, and nipples. You might end up looking healthy and glowing, but you might also seem a little blotchy.

Sinus Congestion: Although your body's overall health has benefited from the improved blood flow, the nasal passages might become highly irritated. In fact, as your blood volume rises, your sinuses and nasal mucous membranes swell, giving you a stuffy nose.

Prenatal Care

By now, you should be getting along well with your obstetrician! You'll likely schedule an appointment once a month throughout the second trimester to make sure everything is proceeding as planned. Here are a few things to anticipate before seeing the doctor.

Tests: There are a ton of them. To make sure you are in top condition, all of the regular diagnostic procedures, including blood tests, urine tests, and blood pressure checks, will be carried out. Also, your weight will be closely monitored as well as the abdomen.

Movement: The first time you should feel the baby move should be around 20weeks. When did you first feel movement in the womb? is something your healthcare practitioner will want to know.

Heartbeat: An ultrasound will be done to see the baby and ensure that everything is progressing normally. You'll be able to hear the baby's heartbeat at this point.

Prenatal Testing: Although it's not required, it's usually a good idea to think about getting prenatal testing done to assess the likelihood of congenital malformations, hereditary disorders, and other issues of the same nature. Blood tests to screen for genetic issues, ultrasounds to check for developmental issues, and more invasive tests like the amniocentesis to check for particular disorders are often conducted testing.

Diet and Exercise

There is no reason why you cannot continue to be active throughout the second trimester if you were active before your pregnancy and during the first trimester, of course with your doctor's approval. To avoid losing your equilibrium, stay away from jarring physical exercises. Your center of gravity shifts significantly as your belly expands, increasing the likelihood that you will fall. Hiking, mountain biking, skiing, and any other activities that put your stomach at risk should be avoided.

Your hunger could seem to be growing. You will need to eat a little bit more (of healthy foods, that is) to maintain a greater calorie intake even though you are not actually eating for two.
For the sake of your child's healthy development, you must maintain your energy levels. To keep those carbohydrates in your system, try eating multiple smaller meals throughout the day.

Development
You're actually cooking now! Every day the baby grows and changes, becoming more and more like a small person. Here is a summary of what the unborn child is doing week by week within the womb.

Weeks 13–15: Although you can't feel it yet, the baby begins kicking and moving all throughout at week 13. The development of the prostate in males and the placement of the ovaries in females make the sex of the newborn more and more obvious. The baby will also begin to grow skin and potentially hair follicles at week 15.

Weeks 16–18: The fetus is now able to clench its fist and exhibit basic facial emotions. At week 17, the body starts to store fat for protection and warmth during labor and delivery. As the ears develop, the baby will be able to hear your heartbeat, stomach rumblings, and loud noises coming from outside the womb.

Weeks 19–21: The baby's skin is now covered in a barrier known as vernix. You are halfway through your pregnancy at this point, and you can probably feel your baby moving. Baby can consume amniotic fluid during week 21 and get nutrition from it.

Weeks 22–24: During this time, your baby will start to explore the world around him or her by touching various objects. It's incredible to think that females have all of their eggs at this moment. At week 23, the skin begins to gradually lose its transparency and the lungs begin to prepare for breathing outside the womb. Baby can now determine if he is upside down or right side up because his inner ear is fully grown. Baby will sleep and wake up at regular intervals.

Weeks 25–27: The baby will continue to use her hands to touch and feel everything around her even though the nerve connections have not yet fully developed. Eyebrows, head hair, and eyelashes are all properly and fully growing. Baby's length will have expanded by at least three times from the end of the first trimester to the end of the second.

Trimester Three
Your fantastic pregnant odyssey is about to come to an end. You can be counting down the minutes till it's over or savoring every second. Every woman has a unique experience.

Symptoms
While many of the bothersome symptoms you experienced at the beginning of your pregnancy have now subsided, you may still feel uncomfortable or develop new symptoms. You should have a sense of what to anticipate from the following.

Swelling: Third-trimester pregnant women frequently experience swollen feet. Your expanding tummy puts pressure on the veins in your legs, causing swelling as the blood returns to them. Other body parts, like the face and hands, may start to swell as a result of all those dilated blood vessels.

Backaches: As your baby grows, your abdomen expands as well, placing significant strain on your lower back. Not to mention the fact that pregnant hormones cause the ligaments holding your bones together to relax. Your back will be more strained as a result.

Varicose Veins: If you have varicose veins, you will detect blue or elevated veins on your body. During pregnancy, the legs tend to show these the most frequently. Blood tends to pool in the legs, resulting in ugly eruptions, as a result of the pelvic veins being somewhat constricted.

Increased Urination: During your last trimester of pregnancy, you should anticipate many trips to the restroom. Baby will put increased pressure on your bladder as she grows, giving you the impression that you need to relieve yourself frequently. Additionally, the pressure will become even more after the baby is born closer to your due date.

Bigger Breasts: They do continue to expand! Pregnant women typically develop 1-3 pounds of breast tissue! Additionally, as your due date approaches, be prepared to start leaking colostrum, the nutrient-rich fluid your unborn child will need to survive for a few days after birth.

Weight Gain: A gain of around 30 pounds is typical throughout pregnancy. While the baby contributes to some of this extra weight, so do a number of other factors, including the placenta, the more blood in your body, increased fat, and fluid retention.

Prenatal Care

As your due date draws nearer, your doctor visits will increase. Expect additional pelvic examinations and general discussion of your cervix's health. Throughout the third trimester, you will also undergo testing for a number of conditions, including

Group B Strep: Some women's rectums or vaginas are home to the bacteria known as Group B Strep. Although it won't hurt you, if the infant is exposed to it at birth, it can lead to a serious infection. If your test results are positive for this bacteria, you'll probably need to take antibiotics throughout delivery.

Anemia: Iron supplements are necessary to raise hemoglobin levels if you are determined to be anemic, which is characterized by a low red blood cell count.

  You'll need to take iron supplements to increase your blood's hemoglobin level. Anemia during pregnancy might result in preterm labor and possibly impaired development.

Diabetes: Gestational diabetes is a type of the disease that exclusively develops in pregnant women. If you are diagnosed, managing the condition with a healthy diet should be possible.

The movement of your infant will also be watched. If your baby is breech, or with its feet down, the doctor may try to turn it using a technique called external version, in which he applies pressure to the abdomen in a specific way to help the baby to turn. A breech infant will almost always require a C-section. You'll probably be invited to visit once every week beginning in week 36 until labor starts.

Fitness and Diet

You should be able to carry on with your workout regimen as usual if everything appears to be in order. Just stay away from anything that can make you lose your balance. Additionally, avoid doing any heavy lifting because it can make you unbalanced and put a lot of pressure on your abdomen.

And keep in mind that you are eating for more than one person, not two! To ensure that you and your baby get all the necessary nutrients, you should slightly increase your caloric intake

Development

It is now on! Inside the womb, the baby is changing and growing quickly. As your due date approaches, read on to learn how your baby is doing.

Weeks 28–30: The baby's eyes are now able to open and close, and you will notice her movements considerably more. Her kicks will become considerably more audible as her bones become harder. From this point on, the baby will also carry on gaining weight, up to a half pound a week.

Weeks 31 to 33: The baby's lungs continue to mature. If he is born at this time, his chances of living are very good. Furthermore, the hair that had been concealing his skin suddenly starts to fall off. Week 33 marks his ability to perceive light, his pupils' contraction and dilate.

Weeks 34–36: The vernix, a white, filmy covering, thickens considerably at this point and may even be still be visible at birth. Baby is likely to move less than usual because his room is getting smaller as he grows. He can now additionally suckle and is presumably putting his head down to get ready to give birth.

Weeks 37-39: Congratulation! At 37 weeks, the baby is full-term. She keeps gaining weight and storing fat, which causes her to be rounded like a baby during delivery. The brain is still growing and will keep growing throughout childhood.

Week 40 has arrived! Your due date has passed, and your child should enter the world at any moment.

Delivery and Labor

It's finally that moment! You suddenly have your first contraction while reruns of a favorite TV show are on. Not to worry! As soon as your contractions are five minutes apart, call the people you need to call, grab your overnight bag, and go to the hospital.

Earliest Stage of Labor

Unless your water bursts or your contractions begin to become regular right away, it may be difficult to pinpoint the precise moment when labor begins. Braxton Hicks contractions may continue until labor actually begins. You might not even notice your contractions at first if they are light.

But if early labor begins, you could feel pain with these contractions. Some women are able to carry on with their daily chores when they are in early labor. In fact, some claim it helps them relax by taking their minds off the next, more strenuous job. The most important thing is to follow your instincts. Take a stroll or a bath.

Additionally, due to the fact that bloody show is frequently present, you'll experience a higher frequency of vaginal discharge. Most likely, you can wait out early labor in the convenience of your own home.

Going to the hospital will be necessary after your contractions become more frequent, but the exact time should be negotiated with your doctor. It is advisable to take it easy during this stage of labor, drink lots of water, and urinate frequently. You need to conserve your energy for the harder parts of labor.

First Stage: Active Labor
Now, contractions increase in frequency and power. From 4 cm at the start of active labor to 10 cm at the conclusion, your cervix continues to dilate. The baby's rectum will likely be compressed as it continues to descend into the pelvis.
On average, you should expect to be in active labor for six hours. To manage the contractions, it could be useful to shift positions, move around, or get down on all fours. You should also make an effort to rest at intervals. Encouragement, practicing breathing exercises and a relaxing massage from your partner can all help you get through this stage. If you want an epidural, now is the time to obtain one.

Second Stage: Transition
You are nearing the end of your labor. Your cervix will dilate from approximately 8 to 10 cm, and your contractions will intensify and become more frequent. You might feel queasy and want to throw up. Additionally, you can start to shiver uncontrollably. The pressure on your rectum will also increase as the baby moves deeper into the birth canal.

Third Stage: Pushing
Time for the show! Now, it's likely that you'll feel the urge to push with each contraction. When your caregiver gives the go-ahead, it's time to push hard and bear down. You'll start to feel pressure on your perineum as the baby moves more down the birth canal. The doctor could advise you to stop pushing at a certain point so the perineum can expand naturally. Tears can be caused by pushing too hard and too quickly.
Now, not much longer. His mouth and nostrils will be suctioned once the baby has crowned and his face has emerged. One by one, the baby's shoulders are delivered, and then it's done! Your child is here now!
For a first-time mother, delivery can take around an hour without an epidural. It may take a little longer with an epidural. Enjoy your baby in these moments while you wait for Stage 3.

Fourth Stage: Delivery of the Placenta
Your uterus will start to contract once more to separate the placenta from the uterine wall after a brief period of rest. When it really separates, you'll be told to gently press. Your uterus will contract after the placenta is delivered, sealing off any exposed blood veins.
You might want to try nursing your baby right now. Simply keep him

close to your breast, even if he isn't ready to latch on just yet. At this stage, we'll deal with any issues or tears. During that period, you can spend quality time with your partner and the baby. You definitely don't want normal doctor visits and other things to interfere during this joyful period.

Chapter 4: Being a Mother

After the arduous hours of labor and delivery, it's time to relax and enjoy your new baby. The pure joy that a child offers is enough to make up for all of the sacrifices, despite the fact that you might not get enough sleep and feel like you're running on empty.

Bringing a baby home
While your body underwent significant changes throughout your pregnancy (and will continue to do so after delivery), your life will also alter significantly now that the baby is here.

New dads can assist by handling domestic chores, changing diapers, and allowing mom to get some much-needed rest. You might even want to slumber together while the baby snoozes. Take advantage of these peaceful moments because it's likely that you haven't had much alone time lately.

At this stage, you should also anticipate visits from family and friends. Everyone will be excited to meet your newborn, but take care not to overexert yourself. When you're worn out and would prefer to rest than mingle, be honest with your family.

Even though you'll probably feel overwhelmed, keep in mind that there are always people who can assist you. Your spouse, family, and friends would be more than happy to help.

Obtaining a "Mom" status

It could seem a little weird to assume this new role as "mother," given that your mother has always been the only mother you've ever known. In the sense that you don't have to suddenly start acting like one, becoming a mother isn't that difficult. It will probably come naturally to most ladies. Naturally, you'll be concerned about your child's welfare and always try to do what's best for them. The abilities required to deal with your child's conduct are learned as they develop, though. The finer points are learnt, not inherited, just like in every other function in life or even in jobs.

Many first-time mothers, as well as many who are already mothers, believe that having children causes them to lose some of who they are or their sense of self. Even though it might feel like way, it doesn't have to be.

It's not a good idea to let a child take over your entire life. You still need items for your profession, love life, and hobbies, among other things. Even if you might not have as much time to dedicate to these activities as you once did, you can still maintain your "old" self.

Postpartum Depression

While many women go through what is known as the "baby blues," a week or so after the baby is born when they feel a little down, postpartum depression is a completely different situation. Postpartum depression affects between 10 and 15 percent of women, and while it is treatable, it is an extremely dangerous condition.

The start of significant mood changes anywhere between one month and one year after the baby is born is referred to as postpartum depression. It requires medical attention and must be treated with the proper therapy and medication because it is considerably more serious than the baby blues.

Causes

The profound hormonal changes that occur after childbirth are thought to be the cause of postpartum depression. Some women simply endure minor mood changes, but others are plunged into severe depression.

Symptoms

PPD has many distinct ways that it can manifest. There are some significant differences even though the symptoms are extremely similar to those of typical depression. the following are typical signs of postpartum depression:

Lethargy.
Hopelessness.

Appetite loss.
A lack of sleep.
Restlessness.
Constant sobbing.
Shifts in mood.
A lack of interest in activities that one once enjoyed.
Disinterest in the infant.
Confusion.
The fear of self-harm.
Fear of harming baby.

Potential Candidates

A family history of the condition makes you more likely to be diagnosed, much like with any mood disorders and cases of depression. Additionally, if you had postpartum depression during a previous pregnancy or had depression prior to becoming pregnant, you are more likely to experience it this time around. The illness can also increase a woman's likelihood of developing in the event of an unhappy or stressful marriage. Women who don't have close friends or family to confide in are more prone to experience depression.

When experiencing postpartum depression, many women may not discuss their thoughts with their spouses or other loved ones because they feel ashamed of their emotions and lack of interest in their infant. There is no need to feel humiliated or guilty, even if it makes sense why a woman might feel this way. PPD is not anyone's responsibility (except for maybe hormones). It is essential that you let someone know if you suspect PPD so they can help you get the right care. If PPD is not addressed, it could worsen or make you sad for a very long time.

Treatments

When you visit your doctor, they will examine you to rule out any physiological issues first. You will next undergo an examination and receive a PPD diagnosis. Once you've been diagnosed, you can get the right care. A combination of medicine and therapy is one of the most popular PPD treatments. Antidepressants can help your brain's chemical balance return, improving your mood and enabling you to once again enjoy life. Women are given the appropriate coping mechanisms during the therapy component.

Many ladies join a support group as well to help each other get through this difficult period with other women who are experiencing the same or comparable things. Women should stick to their treatment regimen until their doctor advises them otherwise.

Psychosis

A tiny percentage of women who have postpartum depression also experience postpartum psychosis. These women's sadness has gotten out of hand to the point that they experience hallucinations, hearing voices, and infant loss fantasies. According to HealthyMinds.org, it is frequently characterized by "command hallucinations to kill the newborn, or delusions that the infant is possessed. "Infanticide" can tragically result from postpartum psychosis. Treatment for mental illnesses is crucial. Lives may be saved.

Your Partner's Capabilities

Sometimes a woman's husband or partner may blame her for having PPD since they don't fully understand what it is. Most of the time, your partner wants to support you and help; he just might not know how. A woman with postpartum depression's partner can take a number of actions to hasten the healing process, such as:

 Be accessible: Many new fathers have overwhelming feelings. However, by being available to your wife, you can be of great assistance to her. Talk freely and pay attention to her sentiments.

 Don't pass judgment: Being critical of your partner's emotions can seriously harm her health. Don't make her feel guilty for being ill; she can't help it. Just be honest.

Assume more responsibility: New mothers often feel overburdened. By keeping the house clean, making more meals, and taking care of the baby more frequently so she can rest, you can assist her in managing it all better.

Keep an eye out for unusual behavior: Complete lack of interest in the infant, or disregard for her own life by the mother of your child, and notify her doctor right away.

Above all things, it's critical to be conscious of your physical and emotional wellbeing. By keeping a close eye on your emotions, you can simply prevent unneeded issues.

Returning to Normal
Everything changes when you have a baby. Even while it sounds cliché, it is true. No matter when you had your child—whether it was last month or ten years ago—having a child imposes a whole new set of obligations on your life. However, once the chaos of having a newborn settles down, you may return to some kind of normalcy in your life.
Being happy requires that you redefine what "normal" looks like in your life. You won't be able to go wherever you want whenever you want anymore. In every choice you make, you must keep your child in mind. You'll be happier if you embrace this sooner rather than later.

Knowing when to ask for assistance might also lighten your load a little. You cannot be expected to care for your child 24 hours a day, 7 days a week, without taking a break for yourself. Every now and then, ask a close friend or family to watch your children so you may take a long bath, read a book, or go out with your partner.

Regaining your pre-pregnancy body is another aspect of returning to normal. Even while you won't get back to your pre-pregnancy weight right immediately, you can start increasing your exercise and reducing your caloric consumption a few weeks after giving birth (of course with your doctor's approval).

Although being a mother is a significant life adjustment, you don't necessarily have to alter your entire way of life. Create time to indulge in your interests and hobbies to keep them alive. Spending time with your partner will help you maintain your romantic relationship. You may decide to go on a date,, watch movies, or just relax at home.

Chapter 5 - Menopause

Being a woman may be a very stressful experience. You've been able to get pregnant since puberty. Your body underwent significant changes, and your emotions might have ranged widely. A life develops inside of you during pregnancy, and as a mother, you spend a lot of time and effort raising this life. You'll now go through menopause as a woman in your late 40s or early 50s, which will bring about yet another shift.
Many people are unaware that the menopausal process is fairly slow. You don't suddenly become infertile after being a lady who can conceive for a few days. It may begin in your 30s and last until your 60s.

Numerous changes, including hormonal, physiological, and even psychological ones, are linked to menopause. Knowing what to anticipate can help you avoid a lot of stress when your body begins to change quickly and you're not sure why.

Symptoms
By referring to them as symptoms, menopause is made to sound like an illness. While it is unquestionably not a sickness, it does have a number of unpleasant indications and symptoms. Menopause symptoms frequently include:

- Decreased fertility
- Frequency of urination.
- Incontinence of the urine.
- Urinary tract infections are more common.
- Burning and itching in the vagina.
- Lessening of vaginal lubrication
- Variable timeframes.
- Sweating at night.
- Inability to have a good night's sleep.
- An increase in facial, chest, or abdominal hair.
- Gaining weight.
- Hair thinning.
- Acne.
- Heat waves.
- Irritability.
- Fatigue.
- A decline in memory.

What Starts the Menopause Process?

Once the ovaries begin to reduce estrogen production, menopause sets in, and your chances of getting pregnant will gradually decline.
Pre-menopause is the name for the initial stage of menopause. Despite the fact that you are still ovulating and capable of becoming pregnant, it consists of menopause's warning signs and symptoms. Your hormone levels drastically fluctuate. Once you have gone 12 months without a period, you enter the second phase. You will spend the remainder of your life in this phase, which is known as post-menopause.

What Might Cause an Early Menopause?

Menopause is a fully natural process; however it might start sooner than usual as a result of surgery or certain medical procedures.
Menopause normally does not begin after a hysterectomy in which just the uterus is removed; however, menopause may begin after a hysterectomy in which the ovaries are also removed. Women who have this surgery do not experience the pre-menopause. Instead, they will start to show signs of menopause and stop bleeding right away. As part of their cancer treatment, radiation-treated women may potentially experience an early menopause.

Options for Medical Treatment

Menopause itself is not a disorder that has to be treated, but the uncomfortable symptoms it might produce can sometimes be managed with certain medical procedures. There are several illnesses that can be treated as well, many of which are more common in postmenopausal women.
- Studies have shown that low-dose antidepressants can lessen hot flashes.
- Non-hormonal medications like Fosamax and Actonel that slow bone thinning and osteoporosis.
- To treat some urinary tract issues and vaginal dryness brought on by menopause, local estrogen is occasionally used.
- Hormone therapy, often known as HT, is the most widely used drug to treat menopause symptoms. Although it can significantly lessen menopause symptoms, the additional estrogen can increase your risk of stroke, heart attack and breast cancer.

Home Remedies

There are numerous things you may do in the comfort of your home to reduce menopause symptoms. They consist of:

Keeping up your sexual activity can help relieve vaginal discomfort during menopause. The dryness and discomfort experienced during sexual activity and during the day can also be lessened by using water-based lubricants.

Consume a diet that is well-balanced and rich in fruits, leafy green vegetables, whole grains, and calcium.

To help squelch those hot flashes, exercise frequently and dress in layers.

Steer clear of anything that seems to trigger hot flashes, such as extremely hot environments, alcohol, or spicy foods.

Learn how to unwind at night using relaxation methods like meditation to get the best possible sleep.

Perform "Kegels" each day. By strengthening the pelvic floor, these workouts help prevent urine incontinence.

Visit your physician frequently. Regular checkups help you feel confident in yourself and enable you to receive any necessary medical care as soon as you require it.

Women must travel a route through life that can be rather difficult, but it is also one that is full of incredible transformations and experiences. We can only fully appreciate the wonder, that is, a woman if we comprehend our bodies and the procedures they go through.

ABOUT THE AUTHOR

Anibaba Omoyemi is a graduate of Communication and Language Art from the prestigious University of Ibadan, Oyo State, Nigeria. She is a freelance writer, teacher and broadcaster. She loves to do a lot of research in order to expose herself to so much knowledge. She is very inquisitive and believes knowing something about everything is very important to equipping oneself. Her inquisitiveness bore this book.